Leadership's Deeper Dimensions: Building Blocks to Superior Performance

Management Series Editorial Board

Your board, staff, or clients may also benefit from this book's insight. For more information on quantity discounts, contact the Health Administration Press Marketing Manager at (312) 424-9470.

This publication is intended to provide accurate and authoritative information in regard to the subject matter covered. It is sold, or otherwise provided, with the understanding that the publisher is not engaged in rendering professional services. If professional advice or other expert assistance is required, the services of a competent professional should be sought.

The statements and opinions contained in this book are strictly those of the author and do not represent the official positions of the American College of Healthcare Executives or of the Foundation of the American College of Healthcare Executives.

Reprinting March 2011

Library of Congress Cataloging-in-Publication Data

Atchison, Thomas A., 1945–
    Leadership's deeper dimensions : building blocks to superior performance / Thomas Atchison.
       p. cm.
    Includes bibliographical references.
    ISBN–13: 978-1-56793-251-5
    ISBN–10: 1-56793-251-7 (alk. paper)
    1. Health services administration—Psychological aspects. 2. Health services administrators—Psychology. 3. Chief executive officers—Psychology. 4. Executive ability—Psychological aspects. 5. Leadership—Psychological aspects. I. Title.

RA971.A878 2005
362.1068—dc22

2005052838

The paper used in this publication meets the minimum requirements of American National Standard for Information Sciences—Permanence of Paper for Printed Library Materials, ANSI Z39.48-1984.♾™

Acquisitions editor: Janet Davis; Project manager: Jane Calayag; Cover designer: Trisha Lartz

Health Administration Press
A division of the Foundation of the
    American College of Healthcare Executives
1 North Franklin Street, Suite 1700
Chicago, IL 60606-3529
(312) 424-2800

Introduction

WORD LIST A

Meaning

Purpose

Achievement

Feeling in control

Making a difference

Being part of something good

A contributing member of a team

Finding joy in the doing

Helping others

Giving more than receiving

Growing

Learning

Teaching

Loving

Clear direction

Celebration

Clear vision

Shared values

Fun

WORD LIST B

Fear

Uncertainty

Doubt

Mistrust

Disrespect

Anxiety

Economic self-interests

Hidden agendas

Personal attacks

Fatigue

Avoidance

Blaming

Lying

Unappreciated

Poor communication

No one listens

No clear direction

Budget-driven decision making

Wishing you could retire or move to another job

Anger

Frustration

Apathy

Think about any conversations you have had in the last two weeks about your workplace. Recall the words you used to describe this place. Were most of the descriptive words you used located on List A or List B? Those who find yourselves using words on List A are leaders with many followers and do not need to read this book. However, you may want to read why the words on List A are so common when you discuss your workplace. Those of you who view List B as most descriptive of your work environment have a title but no followers and may well benefit from the concepts in this book.

My 22 years in healthcare consulting have given me an opportunity to work with some of the finest healthcare leaders in this country. I have encountered very highly paid titled executives who make Nicolo Machiavelli seem like Mother Theresa. The ever-increasing pressures on healthcare executives today seem to delineate, more rapidly than ever before, the difference between true healthcare leaders (those with followers) and titled executives (those who sit in high positions on the healthcare chain of command but have no followers). I have written about these differences in the book *Followership* (Atchison

2004). This book expands on the concepts in *Followership* and explores the *deeper dimensions* of healthcare leadership.

This book is the result of two diametrically opposing experiences I had recently. Last year had been unusual work-wise in that the consulting requests seemed to be bimodal. On the one hand, we were receiving calls from executives who were in deep trouble, typically with physicians. On the other hand, we were hearing from executives who were doing exciting things but needed help in maintaining their momentum. This bimodal pattern occurred at the same time I was rereading Viktor Frankl's (1983) book *Man's Search for Meaning* and Mihaly Csikszentmihalyi's (2003) *Good Business: Leadership, Flow, and the Making of Meaning*.

From these two experiences, a question emerged: Why are some high-ranking people in healthcare able to create a high-performing work environment, and why do others create a toxic work environment? Both Frankl and Csikszentmihalyi suggest that the key to this puzzle is in the word *meaning*. Frankl (1983, 125–26) ". . . considers man a being whose main concern consists in fulfilling a meaning, rather than in mere gratification of drives and instincts... or in the mere adaptation and adjustment to society." He reinforces his core belief about people with a quote from Nietzsche: "He who has a why to live for can bear almost any how" (126).

Csikszentmihalyi (2003, 154) makes the importance of meaning very clear: "If a leader can make a convincing case that working for the organization will provide relevance, that it will take the workers out of the shell of their mortal frame and connect them with something more meaningful, then his vision will generate power, and people will naturally be attracted to become part of such a company."

The stresses in healthcare leadership are essentially the same for both high-performing and low-performing executives. No differences can be explained in terms of the leader's geography, age, gender, amount of experience, or academic preparation and the organization's corporate structure. What are those deeper characteristics that separate high performers from those with serious personnel problems? This book presents one model that relies on the deeper dimensions possessed by healthcare leaders who excite their trustees, physicians, executives, associates, and communities.

The book does not claim to be based on research. This work lays out my subjective interpretation of the current state of healthcare leadership. I hope that it promotes serious discussions and provokes important questions among those who train, develop, hire, and mentor today's and tomorrow's leaders. I welcome challenges to my conclusions. I would also welcome positive stories about how the model I propose, or parts of it, helped in inspiring followers to reach their potential and become high-performing professionals.

REFERENCES

Atchison, T A. 2004. *Followership: A Practical Guide to Aligning Leaders and Followers*. Chicago: Health Administration Press.

Csikszentmihalyi, M. 2003. *Good Business: Leadership, Flow, and the Making of Meaning*. New York: Penguin Books.

Frankl, V. 1983. *Man's Search for Meaning* (Revised and Updated). New York: Pocket Books.

CHAPTER 1

The Basic and New Models of Leadership

The main lesson from these two models is that all leaders balance the inputs and outputs—that is, the tangibles, the intangibles, and the corporate soul.

PART 1: THE BASIC MODEL

A leader without followers is not a leader (Atchison 2004). Healthcare professionals who have titles (also known as titled executives) and control over any number of staff cannot be considered leaders unless their staff are inspired to follow them. The critical (and only) variable in healthcare leadership is the degree of inspiration felt by followers. The critical (and only question) that titled healthcare professionals need to ask is, When I turn around, is anyone there? Titled executives without followers are at best ineffective and, unfortunately, often toxic to the organization's mission. Leaders have followers who are inspired to achieve a vision and who build teams to manage change. This definition explains the dynamic between a leader and his or her followers. The leader-follower relationship is simple to understand but difficult to build. ▶

The Power of Vision

The only reason people follow someone else's lead is that they believe that the leader will take them to a better place—a place that they cannot get to themselves. Therefore, the process of leading others begins with the creation of a destination. This destination must be a place that is better than what currently exists, can be visualized by all involved, and is reachable. Several authors (Atchison 2004; Collins 2001; Schein 1997; Kotter and Cohen 2002) have called this destination a *vision*.

A vision is a short, inspirational statement of where the organization intends to be in the future. The easiest way to understand the power of a vision is to think of it as a probability statement. A vision statement becomes the guideline for the leader and followers, measuring both their actions against the question, Will this behavior increase or decrease the probability that we will achieve our vision? If the answer indicates that the behavior decreases this probability, then the behavior is altered or eliminated. A simple example can be illustrated by a personal vision of losing 30 pounds. The person's vision allows him or her to make a choice between a piece of cake or a stick of carrot; the vision prevents the person from doing anything that will decrease the chance of weight loss.

A vision is the most important factor in inspiring followers, because it is a clear framework for decision-making processes and thus results in follower commitment to its achievement. Leaders know that no one will follow them to yesterday or follow them to mediocrity. Therefore, vision plays a powerful and initial role in bonding leaders and followers.

Values Alignment

The second most critical element that aligns leaders and followers is shared values. Values are beliefs that drive behavior; they are "hard-wired" convictions that guide our decision making. All actions, decisions, conflicts, problems, and complaints about the world around us are anchored in personal values. To a very large degree, our ideas on and responses to opposites, such as Republicans or Democrats and Christianity or Judaism, are predetermined by our hard-wired values.

Leaders understand that the degree to which their values are aligned with those of their followers is a critical element in ensuring followership. The relative position of vision and values (or which should come first—vision or values?) is debatable. I believe that the leader creates an inspiring, directional, and measurable vision and then uses a values-based staff selection process to achieve alignment. However, Jim Collins (2001, 44) in his book *Good to Great* states that leaders must start with the right people: "Get the right people on the bus, get the wrong people off the bus, put the right people in the right seats, and drive the bus." His notion of values first, vision second, however, may be more appropriate to the non-healthcare industry. Healthcare, by the nature of the work, tends to attract professionals with caring values. Therefore, the healthcare leader must first create a vision, then align followers' values to the context of that established vision. In healthcare, the driver (leader) must first figure out where the bus needs to go, select the right people and get the wrong people out of their seats, put the right people in the right seats, and make everyone on the bus sing the same song.

Corporate Culture

Leaders know that it is impossible to motivate anyone, or to demotivate anyone, for that matter. Leaders accept the fact that all people are 100 percent motivated 100 percent of the time. This fact begs the question, What environmental factors unleash the followers' potential, and what environmental factors inhibit or suppress the followers' potential? The organization's corporate culture is the answer.

Corporate culture is the organization's ecosystem, its personality, and its standard of how everyone behaves. Culture is the expression of the core values held by all employees. Think of very successful companies, such as Wal-Mart, GE, Nordstrom, P&G, and Southwest Airlines; their employees live the established core values, delivering consistent performance regardless of location, time of day, or position within the company. All high-performing companies, both within and outside of the healthcare industry, are led by individuals who have followers simply because the followers are inspired by the leader's vision, believe in the corporate values, and work in an environment that unleashes their human potential.

Change Management

Leaders and followers are a powerful force in managing change. The true beauty of leadership lies in the leader's and followers' ability to together create a new, different, and better future. The leader's ability to affect the environment through his or her followers is unique.

The art and science behind change management is not complicated. Its science simply states that all human beings prefer to do things that have the most meaning for them. Therefore, when a follower perceives that the leader wants to change in a direction that is meaningful to the follower, then accepting the change is easy. When the change is understood, is something the follower wants, and makes the follower feel that he or she has some control over the change process, then resistance to the change is not likely. The opposite is true if the follower is kept in the dark and perceives no involvement or control over what is about to take place. In this case, the leader–follower bond is broken.

The art of change management is harder to define. Leaders seem to possess an innate ability to understand the communication requirements of each group of followers and potential followers. The leadership style of Kathy McDonagh, Ph.D., FACHE, CEO of Christus Spohn Health System in Corpus Christi, Texas; Todd Linden, CHE, CEO of Grinnell Regional Medical Center in Grinnell, Iowa; and Pete Delgado, CEO of LAC + USC Healthcare Network in Los Angeles, California, is a joy to watch. These healthcare leaders are able to adjust their styles to the needs of their followers. Their communication style adjusts immediately to the needs of their audience as well. An image for comparison that comes to mind is that of a world-class snow skier, gliding from one turn to another at extreme speeds but always in control.

THE EVOLUTION OF THE BASIC MODEL

The original foundation for all of my writing and consulting is the model (circa 1984) shown in Figure 1.1. Over the years, this model evolved to incorporate the corporate soul (see Figure 1.2).

The main lesson from these two models is that all leaders balance the inputs and outputs—that is, the tangibles, the intangibles, and the corporate soul. The concepts in these two models are still valid and need to be kept in the forefront of all healthcare leaders' decision making. However, today's healthcare climate entails a new level of complexity.

Relationships between management, staff, and care providers are more conflicted, less civil, and more egocentric. Consequently, leaders find it more difficult to inspire followers. This complexity of human relationships forced me to again look deeper into the tangible, intangible,

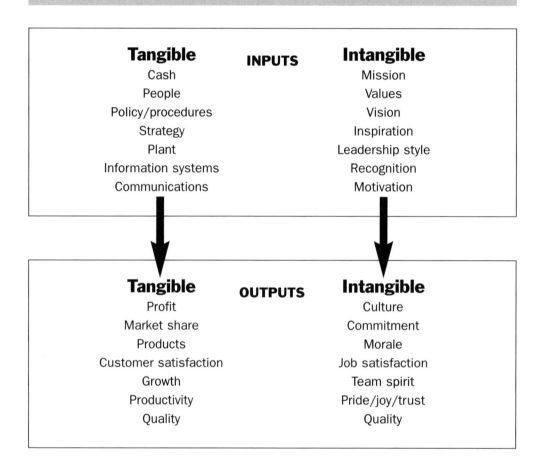

Figure 1.1. Basic Leadership Model

Tangible	INPUTS	Intangible
Cash		Mission
People		Values
Policy/procedures		Vision
Strategy		Inspiration
Plant		Leadership style
Information systems		Recognition
Communications		Motivation

Tangible	OUTPUTS	Intangible
Profit		Culture
Market share		Commitment
Products		Morale
Customer satisfaction		Job satisfaction
Growth		Team spirit
Productivity		Pride/joy/trust
Quality		Quality

and corporate soul model that has served me for so many years.

By taking each piece of the earlier model and applying it to current relationship problems that my consulting practice was hearing about, I discovered the deeper dimensions that underlie today's healthcare leadership problems.

The Deeper Dimensions

The deeper dimensions of leadership are located mainly in the outputs of the corporate soul. Since the mid-1980s, an ever greater emphasis has been placed on the financial aspect of traditional healthcare delivery. Also, a growing number of consultants and stakeholders appear

Figure 1.2. Basic Leadership Model with Corporate Soul

	Tangibles	Corporate Soul	Intangibles
INPUTS	• Cash • People • Policy/procedures • Strategy • Plant • Information systems • Communications	• Meaning • Caring • Giving	• Mission • Values • Vision • Inspiration • Leadership style • Recognition • Motivation
OUTPUTS	• Profit • Market Share • Products • Customer satisfaction • Growth • Productivity • Quality	• Inner peace of purpose • Joy • Pride	• Culture • Followers • Commitment • Job satisfaction • Team spirit • Trust • Quality

to advise executives and boards to ignore their missions in favor of developing and profiting from high-margin services. The most toxic phrase ever stated in healthcare is "no margin, no mission." By placing money in front of caring, healthcare is losing its soul.

Of course, good business practices must support the mission, but the mission should never drive profit maximization. The emphasis on money, market share, production, and profitability has changed healthcare from a "transformational experience to a transactional one," as my good friend Dr. Joe Bujak (2005) states.

The degree of toxicity caused by an overemphasis on money at the expense of mission has significantly eroded the infrastructure that supports the good faith in the organization by the community, the physicians, the nurses, other caregivers, and all other staff. A recent *Modern Healthcare* (2005) article quoted the latest results from the American College of Physician Executives' annual survey. The results indicate that physicians are the fifth most trusted professionals (behind grade-school teachers and pharmacists). In the history of this survey, physicians had always been ranked as the number one most trusted group. The article enumerates many reasons for this fall from grace, each having to do with the public's perception of the economic gains enjoyed by treating physicians.

PART 2: THE NEW MODEL

The new model shows a developmental, hierarchical process to rebuild the critical underpinnings of a successful healthcare organization. At the heart of this model are the deeper dimensions of leadership.

Trust

The most obvious problem in today's healthcare industry is the loss of trust. In my 22 years in the consulting field, I have heard from physicians, nurses, administrators, trustees, and other professionals whose personal experiences in healthcare have critically eroded their trust in others in the field. Several of these discussions ended with these professionals questioning whether they should stay in the industry.

The lack of trust is so pervasive in healthcare today that I made trust the foundation for the rest of the elements in the new leadership model, followed by respect, pride, and joy.

The developmental aspects of this model cannot be overemphasized. Any attempt to establish a sustainable organization without first building trust is a fool's journey. As Dr. Matt Lambert III (2005), FACHE, a well-known physician leader in healthcare, articulates,

"Trust is the foundation of all long-term relationships, yet it is one of the characteristics of leadership that is not discussed enough. Before you ask others to trust you, you must show your faith in them. When one's reputation becomes known in this regard, it is quite gratifying to have people seek you out because they 'heard you can be trusted.' Although it may take years to build a strong relationship, when trust is violated, that bond can be destroyed in an instant. Leaders who lose the trust of others may find it difficult to get a second chance."

Respect

Something strange seems to be happening in healthcare: Physicians, nurses, and other caregivers are viewing each other and, more disturbingly, are being viewed by the communities they serve with more suspicion than respect. Respect begins with simple civility, which should be well supported by high regard for everyone's contributions. Working in healthcare cannot be so difficult that taking time out to give someone a pat on the back for good work becomes impossible.

Pride

A work environment dominated by trust and mutual respect can easily build pride. Focusing on employee pride rather than employee satisfaction is more important. People love to perform at their best and get very excited when they achieve a new level of performance. This excitement is the pride in completing a task or meeting a challenge that pushed them to new and higher levels of performance.

Joy

Confucius says, "Find a job that you love, and you'll never work another day in your life." Like the other three dimensions, joy is a rare commodity in today's healthcare. Staff and professionals who are allowed to apply their skills and experience with a minimum of uncontrolled distractions find that their work brings them joy. The

abundance of workplace regulations, the organization's obsession with short-term financial targets, the short amount of time in which numerous tasks are required to be performed in a day, and the often limited number of qualified and committed staff available to complete the tasks have replaced joy with frustration.

THE SYNERGY FACTOR

The original basic model and several early versions of the new model were reviewed by many friends and colleagues, most of whom are mentioned in the acknowledgments. Their help was invaluable in creating the model I present in this book.

The most important result of our group's discussion is the realization of the concept of synergy. That is, to bridge the difference between the intangible dimensions (trust, respect, pride, and joy) and the tangible realities (clinical quality, patient safety, and financial performance) of organizational performance, synergy is needed (see Figure 1.3).

Synergy is the X factor, or the link that joins the multiple vagaries of the human aspects with the business aspects of healthcare. It is the unique art of leadership, one that establishes and maintains organizational spirit. In Chapter 6,

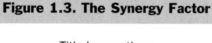

Figure 1.3. The Synergy Factor

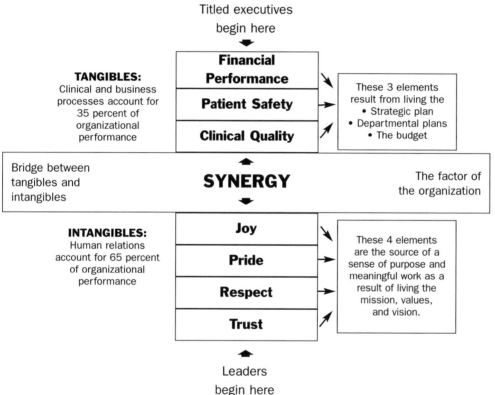

Titled executives
begin here

TANGIBLES:
Clinical and business processes account for 35 percent of organizational performance

Financial Performance

Patient Safety

Clinical Quality

These 3 elements result from living the
• Strategic plan
• Departmental plans
• The budget

Bridge between tangibles and intangibles

SYNERGY

The factor of the organization

INTANGIBLES:
Human relations account for 65 percent of organizational performance

Joy

Pride

Respect

Trust

These 4 elements are the source of a sense of purpose and meaningful work as a result of living the mission, values, and vision.

Leaders
begin here

healthcare leaders who have this X factor are highlighted. Suffice it to say that without this bridge—without creating an organizational spirit—the four intangibles and the three tangibles are seen as discrete entities at best. At worst, the intangibles only come into play during a crisis or conflict.

The model shows that the tangibles rest on the intangibles. The intangibles, or the deeper dimensions, support all tangible gains. Trust, respect, pride, and joy account for 65 percent of organizational performance, while clinical quality, patient safety, and financial performance account for only 35 percent. The tangibles are very important, as they are the fruit of hard labor. However, leaders know that fruit can only grow from healthy seeds, which represent the intangibles.

CONCLUSION

The art and science of leadership is one of the most popular topics in healthcare literature. My previous writings about healthcare leadership have focused on the following critical variables:

1. Leaders have followers. Titled executives, on the other hand, do not inspire followers. Therefore, a title without followers is not leadership.
2. Leaders inspire followers because they have envisioned a better place that their followers cannot reach alone.
3. Leaders select potential followers on the basis of the degree that followers' values align with the organization's core values.
4. Leaders create a work environment, an ecosystem, or a corporate culture that unleashes the human potential of all who participate in the organization's mission.
5. Leaders manage change through other people, involving them in the change process by explaining the reasons for the change. In turn, followers want the positive outcome of the change to occur and feel in control over parts of the change that most affect them.

The remaining chapters discuss the art and science of the deeper dimensions, which provide the psychic income, or the sense of meaningful work, to people who enter the healthcare industry to help others.

REFERENCES

Atchison, T. A. 2004. *Followership: A Practical Guide to Aligning Leaders and Followers*. Chicago: Health Administration Press.

Bujak, J. S. 2005. Personal communication with the author.

Collins, J. 2001. *Good to Great: Why Some Companies Make the Leap and Others Don't*. New York: HarperCollins.

Kotter, J. P., and D. S. Cohen. 2002. *The Heart of Change*. Boston: Harvard Business School.

Lambert, M., III. 2005. Personal communication with the author.

Modern Healthcare. 2005. *Modern Healthcare* 35 (12).

Schein, E. R. 1997. *Organizational Culture and Leadership, Second Edition*. San Francisco: Jossey-Bass.

CHAPTER 2

Trust

Trust takes time, and the time used to build trust must be perceived by the parties involved as meaningful.

Trust is the perception of honesty, openness, and consistency. It takes a long time to create and can be destroyed in an instant. In a *Trustee* article, author Don Berwick (2005), founder of the Institute for Healthcare Improvement, identifies the essential problem with healthcare today: Trust is a rare commodity. The physicians do not trust administration; administration does not trust the physicians; the employees do not trust that they will have jobs for the length of their careers; and, most seriously, the communities are losing trust in the healthcare system. As Berwick (2005, 32) articulates, "Doctors fight administrators; administrators fight Medicaid and Medicare; providers fight transparency; health plans fight each other for market share; and nurses fight health plans. Payers demand measurement, and measurers demand payment. Specialists fight for referrals against which gatekeepers fight."

Sustainable leadership success is impossible without trust, as trust is the foundation for all other intangible and tangible factors that create high performance (see Figure 1.3). In *The Trust Prescription for Healthcare*, author David Shore (2005, 3–4) states that "Trust is the currency of all commerce. Its importance is obvious . . . in fact; it permeates every transaction we make. The more trust exists, the easier it is for everyone to do business and the greater is a country's ▶

prosperity." Shore makes a very important point: Trust is the basis for all positive human interactions. Imagine a world where no trust exists. That world is filled with people who second guess their actions and decisions, are passive aggressive, are manipulative, only pursue personal gains, and avoid the real issues. When suspicion replaces trust in an organization (or society, for that matter), maximizing performance becomes impossible.

CRITICAL VARIABLES OF TRUST

Time

Trust increases as a direct function of meaningful interactions. The two lessons from this fact are (1) that trust takes time and (2) that the time used to build trust must be perceived by the parties involved as meaningful. Chip Doordan (2005), CHE, president and CEO of Anne Arundel Medical Center in Annapolis, Maryland, knows the role of time in the ongoing trust-building process. According to Doordan, "A leader gives oneself the freedom to listen. We spend time together; I listen, you sense the freedom to open up, and we grow together."

In their book, *Leaders: The Strategies for Taking Charge*, Warren

Bennis and Burt Nanus (1985, 153) discuss the most basic fact about trust, time, and the successful leader: "Trust is the emotional glue that binds followers and leaders together. The accumulation of trust is a measure of the legitimacy of leadership. It cannot be mandated or purchased; it must be earned. Trust is the basic ingredient of all organizations, the lubrication that maintains the organization." Investing time to engender trust is the critical success factor in creating a culture based on trust.

History and Perception

The second critical success factor in building trust is the perception of the parties involved. A brief review of the literature (Bracey 2002; Rogers 1999; Annison and Bujak 1998) yields no serious discussion on how an individual's personal history affects his or her perception of others, or how historically based perception predetermines whether trust building will be easy, hard, or impossible for any organization. The role and characteristics of perception and human relations are explored in the book *Leading Transformational Change* (Atchison and Bujak 2001, 52–57).

The fundamental basis of the dynamic between history and

perception (as it relates to creating and strengthening trust) is the concept of perception equals reality. All humans are controlled, to a very large degree, by their previous history with other individuals. When a relationship is based on trust, both persons involved expect an honest, open, and consistent dialog or interaction each time. However, if the relationship is characterized by suspicion and previous negative interactions, then the people involved will predictably expect that the other is not telling the truth, has a hidden agenda, and/or will not follow through.

The notion of "preemptive responses" is one that leaders take very seriously. To demonstrate preemptive response, let us consider a simple everyday task. The next time you open your e-mail or look through your "please call" slips, watch your emotional responses and the sequence of your behavior pertaining to the sender of each message. Your previous history with the sender determines your level of enthusiasm for responding. Who do you call first? Who do you put off as long as possible? Who do you call at 12:05 p.m. because you know that they go to lunch exactly at noon every day?

If you have a long, positive history with the individual identified,

then you are likely to respond quickly and with a degree of excitement. On the other hand, if this person is someone whom you do not trust, then you may delay the response as long as possible or at least prepare yourself for an unpleasant interchange. Trust (and its opposite belief—suspicion) is a function of our history with individuals or groups. Leaders constantly audit their perceptions and try mightily to alter those historical relationships that are currently interfering with progress toward trust.

The relationship between perception and trust can be affected several ways. Of course, the trust–suspicion dynamic begins the first time you meet someone. However, preemptive responses are also controlled by someone's credential (educational attainment, professional training); title (CEO, founder); and other indicators such as race, age, ethnicity, and gender. This suspicion, based on previous experience and stereotypical characterization of others, is a big barrier to trust development.

Honesty is one of the main elements in building trust. Given the many preemptive biases that exist in daily relationships, it is imperative that the parties confront the elephant in the room—that is, mistrust and suspicion. Leaders struggle to understand and deal with their own perceptions and then seek to discover those perceptions in others that interfere with building trust.

In his book, *Good to Great: Why Some Companies Make the Leap and Others Don't*, author Jim Collins (2001) writes about how the most successful leaders "confront the brutal facts." He suggests that when all the right people are in the right places and are focused on the right objectives, then "the real question becomes: How do you manage (lead) in such a way as to not de-motivate people? One of the single most de-motivating actions (a leader) can take is to hold out false hopes, soon to be swept away by events" (Collins 2001, 74). Here, Collins is reminding us that leadership is about inspiring followers, not boosting oneself; leaders must not believe their own press releases. Trust is earned and is a function of the degree that followers and potential followers perceive as honest, open, and reliable. The only way to earn this trust and increase followership is to spend time listening and confronting the brutal facts.

Frequency of Interaction

The fact is trust increases with the frequency of meaningful interactions. Frequency (number and amount of time invested in trust-building activities) is essential. Time can be measured; just audit your calendar to find out how you spend this currency. How many minutes per day do you spend with individuals or groups with whom you wish to build trust? Trust does not happen without personal contact, so it is imperative to come together with others—individuals and groups alike.

Defining "meaningful interactions" in this fact is more elusive. It is possible to increase the frequency of personal contact with others with whom you wish to build trust but still worsen the bond among you. While frequency is a necessary prerequisite to trust building, it is grossly insufficient. The content, context, and behaviors of the parties involved determine whether trust will be increased or decreased. Remember, trust-building sessions are seldom "tabula rasas" (blank pages), wherein everyone comes in without prejudices or biases. Historically based perceptions are ever-present. The first time that a new CEO meets with the chief of staff or chief nursing officer, she is encountering these individuals' perceptions of the last CEO. Therefore, one of the worst methods for building trust is to assure others that "you can be trusted!"

Trust is not a declarative sentence about your own trustworthiness; it is a privilege that your own behavior can earn over a period of time. The amount of time needed to build trust depends on the history of the individuals involved and the perceptions of each of these individuals about one another. The amount of time notwithstanding, the critical success element for all trust building is listening.

THE DYNAMICS OF LISTENING

Listening has many components and layers, and three kinds or levels of listening, which are qualitatively different from one another, are discussed in this section. The three types are as follows:

1. Hearing and reacting (selective listening)
2. Engaging and focusing (active listening)
3. Accepting and supporting (reflective listening)

Hearing and reacting listening does not create trust, is toxic, and, regrettably, is very pervasive. Listening is a lost art in the United States; the discussions on any cable or broadcast talk show will indicate the new shouting-down method of getting differing points of view across. Nowadays, it seems *de rigueur* to find faults or points of disagreement with someone and to focus all energy on these points of greatest disagreements. This is not listening; at best, it is bad debating or destructive polemics. In the United States, there seems to be unwritten rules to a universal game of cynicism and defensiveness— those who find the most faults with someone else or who can shout down opposing ideas, win! This is hearing and reacting, and such behavior will never encourage trust. Such selective and judgmental listening adds to not only mistrust but also enmity.

Engaging and focusing listening may also be called active and validating. This kind of listening assumes that the leader is involved in an active, not reactive, process. Here, the leader must engage the other party by using nondirective techniques. Asking focused questions and paraphrasing are two easy and effective ways to demonstrate that you are interested and engaged in the concerns of the other party. Once the issue that brought the two of you together is clarified and accepted, then the validation process must begin. Trust results from a dialog (give and take) that is perceived as honest, open, and reliable.

Validating is where the best solution is discovered, not dictated. This process is not governed by a focus on the easiest answer or the goal of being liked. Too often, we come up with a solution to just make a problem or issue go away or to make us feel liked by others involved in or affected by the decision. These two factors (quick fix and being liked) are incompatible with engaged and focused listening and are hence barriers to building trust. If driven by these two factors, the leader will come across as superficial and shallow. Leaders build trust with followers because they show genuine concern through engagement and validation.

Accepting and supporting listening is the third level. This is the degree of emotions shared by participants in the dialog. For example, if a nurse comes into your office with tears in her eyes and describes random problems in the emergency department, then your trust-building response is to relate to her emotions, or show empathy toward her feeling of being overwhelmed. The trust-busting response, on the other hand, is to tell her to get over it because life is hard.

This type of listening has a therapeutic component, making people feel safe and accepted for who they are, not just for what they do. In this instance, the challenge for the leader is to allow the follower to express his or her feelings without being sucked into a relationship based on emotion, because sometimes the line between empathy/support and codependency is thin. Be a leader, not an enabler. The key is to respond to the emotional components of the issues and then, as soon as reasonable, steer the discussion toward the second level of listening—engaging and focusing. No matter how emotionally complicated the issue is, at some point it must be fixed. Therefore, trust-building comes from first accepting the individual's feeling as legitimate and then helping that individual gain control of the problem.

Todd Linden (2005), CHE, president and CEO of Grinnell Hospital in Grinnell, Iowa, accepts engaging and focusing listening as one of the best ways that leaders can build trust with followers. According to Linden, "Trust starts with giving people opportunities to spread their wings. It is further developed when leaders bare their souls to followers. Vulnerability helps to put a human face on the boss. Not having all of the answers is important to allowing experimentation."

CONCLUSION

Trust supports all organizational success elements. It is the lubricant that eases tensions among people. Suspicion, enmity, and entropy exist where trust does not. Healthcare organizations without a foundation of trust are very toxic and will destroy all tangible efforts to build sustainable organizational growth, viability, and quality improvement. Trust increases in proportion to the increase in meaningful interactions. Frequency of interactions is a very important prerequisite to trust building. The second prerequisite is the quality of these frequent meetings—the operative word here is *meaningful*.

The degree of meaning as perceived by the follower is defined by the leader's listening skills. Titled executives are known for their selective and judgmental listening, and they often view their followers as economic units that must be pushed to achieve organizational goals. Such executives do not consider the problems that their followers bring up as important. In fact, titled executives seem to enjoy finding fault, taking pride in showing others their weak (and how weak) points. They select, judge, and criticize, and they never listen to understand.

Leaders, on the other hand, listen at the most appropriate level. They seldom get caught up in the polemics of an issue; they listen to understand. They believe that followers are more than economic units and put people before profits, a leadership philosophy clearly expressed by Linden (2005): "It starts with leaders looking deeper into the individual abilities and personalities: What are the skills people have learned? What are the God-given talents the person was born with and developed over time? And, finally, what are the interests that each person or team enjoys?" This perspective illustrates two levels of listening: engaging and focusing and accepting and supporting.

REFERENCES

Annison, M., and J. S. Bujak. 1998. *Trust Matters: How Doctors, Board Members and Health Care Executives Can Work Together Effectively*. San Diego: The Governance Institute, The Medical Leadership Forum.

Atchison, T. A., and J. S. Bujak. 2001. *Leading Transformational Change: The Physician-Executive Partnership*. Chicago: Health Administration Press.

Bennis, W., and B. Nanus. 1985. *Leaders: The Strategies for Taking Charge*. New York: HarperCollins.

Berwick, D. 2005. "The Importance and Paucity of Trust in Today's Healthcare System." *Trustee* 58 (4): 32.

Bracey, H. 2002. *Building Trust: How to Get It! How to Keep It!* Taylorsville, GA: HB Artworks, Inc.

Collins, J. 2001. *Good to Great: Why Some Companies Make the Leap and Others Don't*. New York: HarperCollins.

Doordan, C. 2005. Personal communication with the author.

Linden, T. 2005. Personal communication with the author.

Rogers, R. W. 1999. *The Psychological Contract of Trust: Trust Development in the 90's Workplace*. Pittsburgh, PA: Development Dimensions International.

Shore, D. A. 2005. *The Trust Prescription for Healthcare*. Chicago: Health Administration Press.

EXERCISE: Trust Inventory

Rate yourself (or have your staff evaluate you) on the following items.
(5 = strongly agree; 4 = agree; 3 = sometimes agree; 2 = disagree;
1 = strongly disagree)

1. I am approachable when others have a concern or issue.

2. I encourage honesty and open communication to flow from any
direction.

3. I listen nonjudgmentally regardless of whether the information is good
or bad.

4. I behave consistently.

5. I show interest and concern for others regardless of their position
or power.

6. I meet frequently with my staff even if there is no specific problem to
solve.

7. I make hard decisions about people, processes, and programs that are
ineffective.

8. I show genuine respect for others' knowledge, skills, and contributions.

9. I keep my promises.

10. I explain decisions nondefensively.

CHAPTER 3

Respect

Respect thrives in an environment in which performers are acknowledged for their good work.

Respect is another leadership dimension that supports sustainable growth, viability, and continuous quality improvement. My work in healthcare consulting continues to reinforce the notion that respect is a rare commodity. Many patients do not respect their physicians, nurses, and other caregivers, and many healthcare professionals do not respect each other. This mutual disrespect seems to be a worsening trend. Simple gratitude is a powerful antidote to this downward spiral.

No human feeling is more important to give and more pleasant to receive than basic respect. Dr. Mike Coyle (2005), vice president of medical affairs at Abrazo Health in Phoenix, Arizona, states, "I believe sincere thanks, delivered personally and publicly, best demonstrates my respect for my colleagues." At the risk of seeming banal, I would argue that the rule of common sense and the golden rule go a long way in improving respect within the healthcare field and the people it serves.

Scott Foresman Advanced Dictionary (1997, 940) defines respect as ". . . consideration for someone or something of recognized worth. Respect implies recognition and esteem of worth with or without liking. . . ." This definition emphasizes the intangible significance of respect in organizations. Pete ▶

Delgado (2005), CEO of LAC+USC Healthcare Network in Los Angeles, anchors his leadership in the following philosophy:

> ". . . we are in the people business, [of] people taking care of people. We need more passion in the people business. We are rich in opportunities to make a difference in so many peoples' lives. We need to celebrate this unique opportunity as often as possible."

Delgado has taken this basic personal leadership philosophy and created the "Passionate Performance" reward, a system that compensates staff. He believes that this system is one way, and very powerful at that, to show respect to those who live the hospital's caring values. Delgado is committed to the belief that "It is so important that there are leaders modeling behaviors that show respect for our employees."

POSITIVE ACKNOWLEDGMENT

Respect thrives in an environment in which performers are acknowledged for their good work. Think about the times you felt most and least respected. Typically, people feel most respected when they receive positive feedback from those they hold in high regard. For example, a senior executive stops you in the hallway to compliment you on your high-quality performance mentioned in a patient's letter. One of your peers is standing next to you and says, "I'm glad she commented on your performance. Your work habits have always helped me understand how best to perform. I'm glad you're getting the recognition you deserve." This whole dialog takes less than two minutes, only two out of approximately 500 minutes in a given workday. However, the respect you feel from this two-minute recognition break is immeasurable.

A concept called "positive behavioral contagion" can result from an encouraging comment, such as in the example above. Positive behavioral contagion is the idea that when someone receives recognition, that person is much more likely to return the favor and positively acknowledge someone else. This contagion then creates a cascade or snowball effect, building momentum as recognition moves from one person to another.

Compare this to feeling disrespected. For example, you have led your team to a new high in patient satisfaction, showing a 50 percent increase on your unit over the previous year's data. The vice president presents these data at an all-staff meeting and then quips, "It's about time you and your staff earned your excessive paychecks!" The destructive effect of this kind of statement is immeasurable.

The point here is that, once trust is established, respect is the second most important intangible that supports organizational viability. It is created by positive rewards and recognition, which result in the receiver feeling valued. Insensitive and negative feedback ignores the hard work and contributions of people and often results in their demotivation, hostilility, and strong desire to quit.

CONNECTION BETWEEN RESPECT AND TRUST

Let's examine the two examples of a positive and a negative feedback given above through the first intangible dimension in our sustainability model —trust. Imagine that the positive comment is delivered by someone you trust. Your feeling of being respected then becomes even more valuable and increases your motivation. However, if the same comment is delivered by a person whom you mistrust, you are likely to be suspicious. You might even think that the person has a hidden agenda, is being manipulative, or just got back from a leadership seminar where he or she learned that positive feedback is a powerful motivator. Notwithstanding the actual words spoken, the impact of a positive feedback is dependent on the degree of trust you have in the person giving it.

This fact is also operative in the negative feedback example. Hearing, "It's about time you and your staff earned your excessive paychecks!" from someone you have worked with for years and trust greatly may not have as corrosive an impact on you as it would if you hear it from someone you do not trust. If the speaker is a trusted colleague, you may easily think that he or she is only joking through the actual compliment. Even if the statement does not sound right to you, you most probably would give the speaker the benefit of the doubt, because you trust that he or she would not say anything to embarrass you in front of others. That is, you would reason, "He really didn't mean what he said. He's under a lot of pressure these days."

In other words, the amount of respect created by a recognition or reward event is determined, to a very great amount, by the perception of trust the receiver has in the giver. Once again, trust is the foundation of all tangible and intangible factors in creating a sustainable, viable environment.

REWARDS VERSUS RECOGNITION

People feel respected when they receive a reward or are recognized for their contributions to success. A significant difference exists, however, between rewards and recognition. Recognition is noncontingent, while rewards are contingent. When we recognize someone, we are noticing or acknowledging the person for any number of reasons, many of which do not have anything to do with their contributions. Whereas when we reward someone, we are compensating the person for a specific accomplishment—for exceeding expectations, for example.

For example, healthcare organizations spend a lot of time and money on recognizing events such as birthdays, longevity at or retirement from work, attendance,

and various holidays. Absolutely nothing is wrong with these recognition events, because they are celebrations that promote team unity and communicate to people that they are valued. But such recognitions are not directly tied to organizational performance; it has nothing at all to do with achievement. Do you think that everyone who received a longevity pin was an equal contributor to the organization's quality, safety, and patient satisfaction goals? Because recognition is a noncontingent, feel-good, and celebratory occurrence, its impact on making people feel respected is nowhere near as powerful as that for reward systems.

Rewards are contingent consequences. If a person meets or exceeds a target, then he or she receives a benefit that would not have been available otherwise. Rewards are completely objective; they are binary—that is, they are either hit or missed. An understanding of human behavior is necessary to completely appreciate the objective component of rewards.

Behavior

Behavior has three characteristics: observable, measurable, and repeatable. Behaviors are different from feelings, attitudes, and emotions, as these three cannot be observed but must be intuited. Behaviors are objective, while feelings, attitudes, and emotions are subjective. For example, think of a person who comes 10 minutes late to a meeting. This behavior is observable, measurable, and repeatable. Compare this behavior to a feeling, attitude, or emotion, which is speculative, is subjective, and has little value in organizational change. For example, a late arrival can be taken personally, creating a feeling—"The late person doesn't care about our meeting." A late arrival can inspire an attitude—"The late person is self-centered." A late arrival can stir up emotion—"The late person is probably experiencing guilt about being late."

I continue to be amazed at the amount of time people waste on speculating about other's feelings, attitudes, and emotions. Many discussions about the level of motivation, morale, and commitment of physicians, nurses, and other staff are based on absolute speculation. Imagine if we discussed finances with the same degree of subjectivity and speculation, relying on incomplete or no data. Such lack of specificity would never be considered valid in finance. However, in organizations it is common for senior management

and executives to play psychiatrist, interpreting practices by using their own understanding of what people want and feel.

The lesson here is simple: Behavioral specificity is the only standard that should be used in determining human performance. If the behavior cannot be seen, measured, and repeated, then the behavior is merely a guess and must not be used as a basis for rewards. Behaviors are either desirable or not desirable. Appropriate behaviors are rewarded, while inappropriate ones are not and may even result in negative consequences. This concept of behavioral specificity is critical to the development of an effective reward program.

Again, speculation is never applied to financial matters, which are also binary—financial goals are either achieved or fallen short on. When a variance in the budget is noted, then a gap analysis is used to determine the problem and to find ways to narrow the gap. The same logic must be used for behaviors. Leaders should create a "behavior budget." This budget includes behaviors expected from people and the frequency that they should be displayed per day. Once this behavior budget is in place, a behavioral gap analysis should be done to improve the frequency of desirable behaviors and reduce (or eliminate) undesirable ones. A reward system is effective in increasing the frequency and duration of those behaviors that are consistent with the corporate culture.

REWARD OPTIONS: MONEY VERSUS MOUTH

Money, as it relates to motivating high performance, is very misunderstood and complicated. It is a terrible motivator, only effective in two environments and can be a major demotivator in general.

Using money as a reward can be successful in an environment where that incentive is perceived as fair. However, perceived fairness is an elusive concept, as it relies on opinions of individuals, who although may belong to the same group have, by nature, varying views about what is fair in terms of their contributions. The second environment in which money as a reward can thrive is where there is unpredictability and variation—that is, people do not know when and how much they will get rewarded. This idea is similar to the incentive people have to go to Las Vegas or other gambling sites, or how these places are engineered. People place bets because of the probability that they will win some money or even the jackpot—the reward for playing is different each time. Similarly, staff show appropriate behavior for a duration of time because of the possibility that they will get rewarded. This type of environment is F.U.N.—focused, unpredictable, and novel—and encourages good work toward rewards. Money only motivates when it is perceived as fairly deserved. It also motivates when its arrival cannot be predicted in terms of when and how much.

Money is actually a demotivator when it is expected—that is, when it becomes an entitlement. One of the silliest statements titled executives make is, "I don't know why they don't perform better; they're being paid!" Note that a paycheck is not a motivator; it is seen as entitlement—that is, staff show up to earn their check, regardless of how well or poorly they perform during the course of the workday. They are entitled to receive the paycheck, and this attitude and mind-set are very corrosive to creating respect. If you do not believe this fact, randomly short someone's paycheck by $1.00. Then count the nanoseconds until the phone rings and the affected person demands to know where his or her dollar went.

Money also demotivates when the amount is perceived as too low or even when too high. When a person receives money that is less than expected, he or she feels disrespected. When a person receives a sum that is excessive, he or she may stop performing at a high level or displaying appropriate behavior so as to protect his or her turf, for which rewards are plenty.

A better (and cheaper) way to engender respect is by "mouth management." Mouth management, as I have termed the concept, is quite simple: Watch what you say all the time. All of us should use our mouth less for speaking about ourselves and corporate objectives and more for creating meaningful work. Leaders show respect and create meaning in work by educating their staff about specific behaviors that improve the lives of those they serve.

CONCLUSION

Imagine a work environment in which respect is a daily occurrence, where mutually trusting individuals seek out opportunities to reward and recognize each other. Respect is a very important, but unfortunately often ignored, motivator of high performance. The negative consequences of feeling disrespected are measurable. Medical errors, high turnover rates, low levels of performance, labor action, and conflicts among care groups are but a few of these consequences.

Conversely, staff who feel respected look for opportunities to perform at a high level because they are aware that they will be recognized and rewarded for their good work. Respected staff are not motivated by fear or guilt but by desire to do the best for their patients and customers at all times. Respected professionals are qualitatively better performers than professionals who feel disrespected, regardless of skills or experience.

Money management and mouth management are two ways to increase respect within the organization.

REFERENCES

Coyle, M. 2005. Personal communication with the author.

Delgado, P. 2005. Personal communication with the author.

Scott Foresman Advanced Dictionary. 1997. Upper Saddle River, NJ: Pearson Education.

EXERCISE: Respect Inventory

Rate yourself (or have your staff evaluate you) on the following items.
(5 = strongly agree; 4 = agree; 3 = sometimes agree; 2 = disagree;
1 = strongly disagree)

1. I am known for showing gratitude to my peers and staff.

2. I schedule time daily to find staffs who behave the way we wish everyone behaved.

3. My associates know the specific behaviors that are most desirable.

4. Our orientation process stresses the importance of caring for others.

5. I treat others the way I would like to be treated.

6. I am perceived as fair.

7. Behaviors that are inconsistent with our corporate culture are dealt with immediately.

8. Behaviors that reflect our corporate culture are rewarded immediately.

9. Our recognition practices are enjoyed by all.

10. We have training programs in "mouth management."

CHAPTER 4

Pride

Pride is the result of meeting meaningful challenges.

Too much time and money is spent on employee satisfaction, and too little time and money is spent on employee pride (Atchison 1999; 2003). A 2003 article entitled "Exposing the Myths of Employee Satisfaction" addresses this point:

Healthcare work environments, in most cases, are very stressful. The constant focus on budgets; the pressures from the government, payors, and JCAHO; and staff shortages will not disappear overnight—they may even get worse. Such issues should not be an excuse for creating a toxic work environment wherein good and caring people are too stressed to care about others. And sending those . . . to a mandatory customer service class can only make the problem worse. . . . As leaders your goal should be to cultivate employee pride. Believing you can improve employee satisfaction and performance without pride is an illusion and a grand myth (Atchison 2003, 24).

In his book, *Why Pride Matters More Than Money*, author Jon Katzenbach (2003, 23) defines pride as ". . . the emotional high that follows performance and success." Katzenbach expands on the notion given in Chapter 3 that money plays a very limited role in improving organizational performance: ▶

Perhaps money and what it buys motivate you to excel at your job. But think for a moment about the exhilaration that you feel when a customer or client says that you saved the day for them by getting a critical product delivered when all others had failed. Or recall when one of your colleagues praised you strongly in front of your work group for winning over a difficult customer, thereby enabling them to meet their sales target; or when a respected superior singled you out as a role model of how others should deal with unexpected problems. Those feelings of pride are intrinsic to what you do, how you do it, and with whom you do it; they have little to do with money. More important, such feelings of pride are institution-building rather than self-serving. And, in most cases, they motivate people to excel far more effectively than money or position (Katzenbach 2003, 71).

The successful accomplishment of a difficult goal is a major, if not the key, contributor, to feeling pride in the work being done. Asked how she promotes pride in her organization, Vicki Briggs (2005), president and CEO of Baptist Montclair Medical Center in Birmingham, Alabama (previously president and CEO of Longview Regional Medical Center in Longview, Texas), turned to her staff at Longview Regional for answers. According to Briggs's assistant: "[Vicki] engenders pride by creating reasonable challenges, by assessing the person's capabilities and then giving them opportunities to excel and grow in their job. [She] raises the bar from time to time so that the expectations get greater but still attainable" (Harding 2005). Another staff member, an assistant director of human resources, adds that pride can be encouraged by "asking for employee input. . . . This creates a personalized challenge to work toward our hospital values and participate in a positive outcome" (Hardan 2005). A nurse manager at Longview believes pride is created in the workforce through "creating committees to help change what needs to be changed. [Vicki] gives us a chance to voice our input and allow us to use our own problem-solving skills" (Sobey 2005).

In the past, pride is one of the intangibles pervasive in healthcare. A nurse, physician, and even the hospital accountant not only took pride in their work but were also given a certain cache for the roles they played in the organization. Today, pride is absent for many healthcare professionals and in many healthcare delivery entities. Worse, work pride is not even considered as an important factor and is integrated into many strategic imperatives such as employee recruitment and retention, physician relations, reducing costs, creating new lines of business, and improving patient care and safety. One reason that pride is so rare in today's healthcare environment is that the two building blocks to creating and building pride in the workplace are absent: trust and respect (see Figure 1.3).

THE CHALLENGE FACTOR

Pride is the result of meeting challenges. To achieve pride, however, the challenges (1) must be meaningful and (2) must be within the capacity of the individual responsible.

Meaningful Challenges

Meaningful challenges are those that demand the individual responsible to apply his or her own skills and talents. A challenge, by definition, is something that is difficult, something that pushes the individual to levels that he or she has never reached before. Some challenges are "stretch goals"—objectives that may not be as feasible to reach or are out of the usual capability range. Rick Breon (2005), FACHE, president and CEO of Spectrum Health in Grand Rapids, Michigan, believes that his organization creates pride by setting "high expectations that drive the achievement of an aggressive vision."

Such stretch goals or high expectations create an acceptable degree of personal angst and self-doubt among those who are responsible for the challenge. This anxiety is essential in that it pushes people to work better and harder. Because of the tremendous energy, focus, and efforts required by such an initiative, those responsible feel pride, especially when the goal is attained. Not many people can feel proud of completing a project that is easy or average and that is below their skill level. No one ever brags about being average.

The two variables of a meaningful challenge are psychic equity and aligned values. Psychic equity is an individual's personal stake in the goals because he or she has participated in their development. Many years ago, Dr. Paul (2005), a physician at Rush Presbyterian St. Luke's Medical Center in Chicago, told me an acronym that typifies the main reason that people tend to remove themselves from change projects—NIH, as in Not Invented Here. This acronym is a reminder that all parties involved in any challenge must feel that they have contributed to establishing the goals and finding solutions. The listening techniques described in Chapter 2 can be useful in creating psychic equity.

Aligned values means that the individual's personal beliefs are reinforced as a result of the successful accomplishment of the challenge. This values alignment is critical because the individual will tolerate the level of anxiety brought on by the challenge if his or her values are manifested in the task at hand. Asking people to push themselves (to go the "extra mile") in areas that run counter to their personal beliefs will always fail and will yield creative excuses for why the challenge was not met.

Imagine that the chief nursing officer has engaged the staff in a challenge to increase patient satisfaction by 50 percent in one year. Two teams of nurses in two different units will attempt to meet this challenge. One group of nurses has the following hierarchy of values (or reasons, in order of importance, to come to work):

1. Friendship
2. Being liked
3. Conflict avoidance
4. Quality of care
5. Patient satisfaction

The second group of nurses has the exact opposite hierarchy of values:

1. Patient satisfaction
2. Quality of care
3. Conflict management
4. Being liked
5. Friendship

Judging from these values, which nursing group is more likely to achieve the goal, and which group is more likely to give creative rationalizations about why the goal cannot be achieved? Creative rationalizations are never based on actual performance; they are merely the consequence of incompatible values. Staff, individually or as a group, whose values are not aligned with the values of their respective challenges will fail and never accept accountability.

Challenges Within the Capacity of the Individual

The second characteristic of a challenge is that it must be within the capacity of the individual. Capacity is a simple concept but is left out of most discussions on organizational improvement. The absence of capacity from the planning cycle may be explained by two pervasive myths in healthcare:

1. All staff are intellectually and emotionally equal.
2. All staff need to perform at higher levels is the right motivation.

The first myth explains the existence and proliferation of one-size-fits-all educational programs, toward which organizations spend millions of dollars each year. These programs are usually mandatory for all staff, with management under the belief that if each person receives the same amount and type of education, then one will equally learn how to move toward the desired goal. This myth does not make sense at even the most basic level. Human beings are so different from each other that one educational approach cannot possibly work for all. There is no magic bullet in educating and training staff, and expecting staff to be on the same intellectual and emotional levels when it comes to learning is a waste of time.

The second myth is that all staff will up their motivation to achieve the challenge when the right incentive is in place. Human motivation is a very complex combination of science and art. A simple but true observation is that people are motivated best in environments where they feel trusted, respected, proud of their work, and joyous.

LEADERSHIP PORTFOLIO PROCESS

Kathy McDonagh (2005), Ph.D., FACHE, president and CEO of Christus Spohn Health System in Corpus Christi, Texas, instills pride among the staff using the organization's Leadership Portfolio Process (see Figure 4.1 for the Leadership Portfolio Form). With permission from Christus Spohn, we have reproduced this process below.

The Process
- This comprehensive process was announced at Christus Spohn's joint leadership team meeting.
- Directors were instructed to complete the form.
- Directors were asked to identify their educational level and

Figure 4.1. Leadership Portfolio Form

Employment History

Associate name_____

Job title_____

Location_____

Length of service_____

Length of time in current position_____

Education

Current education_____

Education requirement effective 2008_____

On track to accomplish educational requirement _____

Certifications

Professional certifications held_____

Satisfaction Scores

Recent associate satisfaction scores_____

Recent patient satisfaction scores_____

Leadership Rating

A Role model performance—keep up the good work

B Solid performance—some developmental improvements needed

C Not performing at appropriate leadership level—90-day development plan to follow
   summary of discussion

Associate signature _____ Date_____

Supervisor signature_____ Date _____

Source: Reprinted with permission from Christus Spohn Health System, Corpus Christi, Texas.

determine whether they met, or would meet by 2008, the new educational requirements—by 2008, all directors must achieve a bachelor's degree, and all system service directors must earn their master's degree.

- The form was then forwarded to the direct respective executive to complete the Leadership Rating section.

- Directors were rated A, B, or C, according to the following:
  - Role model performance—keep up the good work
  - Solid performance—some developmental improvements needed
  - Not performing at appropriate leadership level—90-day development plan

The Discussion

- A one-on-one discussion was conducted between each director and his or her executive within a two-week period.

The Results

- We had approximately
  Rated A—20 (10 percent)
  Rated B—160 (80 percent)
  Rated C—20 (10 percent)

- This clearly provides us much room for improvement as we strive to meet our goals to excellence.

Timing and Focus

- The Leadership Portfolio Process was completed separate from the performance evaluation.

Leadership Portfolio Timing

- This worked well . . . as we introduce the process with a rollout of significant salary increases for director-level positions.

- "A" players received salary increases to market. "B" players' salary increase was capped at 25 percent. "C" players received no increase, but were eligible for market adjustment upon satisfactory completion of a 90-day work plan. (Increases were not retroactive.)

This process works because it embodies the critical factor in building pride: It provides meaningful challenges that push the staff or professional to perform at a higher level but does not expect the person to do more than what he or she is capable of doing.

CONCLUSION

Pride is a powerful and contagious motivator. People who are proud of their work and their employers spend a lot of time sharing stories about successes that they both had a hand in. Leaders help each professional create a personal development plan that pushes these employees to new levels of performance. Although initially these stretch programs can cause a lot of anxiety, they ultimately become exciting and rewarding once they become part of the culture of high performance. Starting a leadership portfolio process, such as the one developed at Christus Spohn Health System, is a good step forward. However, such a process is a waste of time without first engendering trust and respect among leaders and staff alike; in fact, doing so will cause untenable fear, anxiety, and doubt throughout.

REFERENCES

Atchison, T. A. 1999. "The Myths of Employee Satisfaction." *Healthcare Executive* 14 (2): 18–23.

———. 2003. "Exposing the Myths of Employee Satisfaction." *Healthcare Executive* 18 (3): 20–26.

Breon, R. 2005. Personal communication with the author.

Briggs, V. 2005. Personal communication with the author.

Hardan, T. 2005. Personal communication with the author.

Harding, R. 2005. Personal communication with the author.

Katzenbach, J. R. 2003. *Why Pride Matters More Than Money: The Power of the World's Greatest Motivational Force*. New York: Crown Business.

McDonagh, K. 2005. Personal communication with the author.

Paul, H. A. 2005. Personal communication with the author.

Sobey, L. 2005. Personal communication with the author.

EXERCISE: Pride Inventory

Rate yourself (or have your staff evaluate you) on the following items.
(5 = strongly agree; 4 = agree; 3 = sometimes agree; 2 = disagree;
1 = strongly disagree)

1. I have a sense of loyalty to this company.

2. I identify with this company.

3. I think about the future of this company.

4. I regret that I chose to work for this company.

5. I do extra work here because I want this company to succeed.

6. I feel that I share in the success and failure of this company.

7. I feel a sense of ownership in this company.

8. It would take very little for me to move to another company.

9. I take pride in being part of this company.

10. I am challenged often to achieve more.

Note: Any indicator less than 4.0 needs to be addressed.

CHAPTER 5

Joy

Feeling joy at work is the result of both self-reflection and the culture of the organization.

So far, we have learned that the four deeper dimensions are developmental and hierarchical—that is, each is founded on another. This means that trust must be established before respect can be created, and trust and respect must be present before pride can form. One point about the dynamics of these deeper dimensions that we have not discussed yet is that the first can be viewed more subjectively than the one after it. This means that trust is the easiest to observe and measure, but respect is less discernible, and pride is even more subjective than the last. The fourth and highest dimension—finding joy in the work—is the most subjective and therefore the most difficult to observe and measure.

Dr. Matt Lambert (2005), FACHE, senior vice president for clinical operations at Elmhurst Memorial Hospital in Elmhurst, Illinois, shares his perspective on joy that reflects the national trend toward this view:

"Healthcare should be joyful work, and it is sad that there exists so much angst among employees, executives, nurses, and physicians. We need to remember ▶

how unique this opportunity is. The very first and last moments of existence of many of our fellow human beings are shared with us. No other profession can say that. But there are a number of barriers in our current system that negatively impact this most personal of human experiences. Leaders can do a great deal to improve patient care by eliminating such obstacles and keeping the patient at the center of all we do. Smoothing the way will do a lot to bring fulfillment and meaning back into our daily efforts."

According to Lambert, joyful work involves a barrier free, values-driven behavior focused on the mission of patient care.

Feeling joy at work is the result of both self-reflection and the culture of the organization. In determining what incites this feeling in yourself, you should recognize what you find enjoyable. When was the last time that the joy of doing a task was so powerful that you were suspended in or taken by it? Was it when you helped save a life in the emergency room? Or when you developed and implemented a program that proved beneficial for all involved? What aspect of your personal life has the greatest meaning or purpose? Is it family, a hobby, or a sport? Mihaly Csikszentmihaly (1994, 5) discusses the conditions necessary for "joyful involvement" in his book *The Evolving Self:* ". . . explore the forces of the past that have shaped us and made us the kind of organisms we are . . . and propose approaches to life that improve its quality and lead to joyful involvement. . . ."

The culture of the organization is the other half of the joyful work equation. Leaders must allow and promote opportunities for staff to think about the importance of their contributions and must maintain a corporate culture in which peoples' values, aspirations, attitudes, and expectations are fulfilled. This is no easy task for leaders, but a task worthy of the difficulties.

CREATING A JOYFUL CORPORATE CULTURE

The first step in creating a culture wherein everyone can experience joyful involvement is to convert the values of the corporate culture into actionable behaviors. The elements and dynamics of such a corporate culture are not discussed here but are defined and explored in my other publications (see Atchison

1990; 2001; 2002; 2004; Atchison and Bujak 2002). Converting values to behaviors can be done in several different ways, two of which are trait analysis and tabula rasa.

Trait Analysis

Trait analysis only deals with behaviors. As you may recall from Chapter 3, behaviors are (1) observable, (2) repeatable, and (3) measurable. For example, talking is a behavior and so are smiling and making eye contact. However, wanting to talk is an attitude, while being happy is an emotion.

The process of trait analysis begins by posing to a small group of high-performing staff this question: Who is currently behaving the way you wish everyone to behave? The participants are then asked to write down the names that immediately come to mind. Round-robin identification of the names can then determine the most ideal individuals (or those mentioned on people's list the most times). Each person's name is written on a flip chart—one name per page. Then under each name, the behaviors shown by the chosen person are listed.

Once the behaviors of the chosen performers are listed, they are ranked according to how they reflect the values of the culture and how they help to maintain the values of this culture.

The final ranking can now be used as a basis for behavioral interviewing, selection, promotion, and performance evaluation. An article in *Healthcare Executive* discusses the contribution of behavioral interviewing in improving organizational performance (May 2005). The key to using behaviors as a decision tool is to specify the values on which behaviors can be based.

Tabula Rasa

The tabula rasa, or blank sheet, method of converting values into behaviors has the same goal as trait analysis—to reveal the most ideal behaviors for the established corporate values. Using tabula rasa, however, is less threatening because it does not rely on naming specific people. Trait analysis can sometimes produce anxiety for those asked to be involved in the process because they are forced to talk about certain employees while leaving others out.

The tabula rasa process begins, once again, with a small group of high-performing staff. They are then asked to imagine that no healthcare delivery system exists in their community and to visualize that they are responsible for creating a high-quality system from the ground up. These staff are then directed to focus on the kinds of physicians, other clinical professionals, and support staff that they will employ for their start-up organization. Then, the group is instructed to list the five behaviors that they will want from the staff they plan to recruit and hire to care for their patient population. The answers are then listed on a flip chart for everyone to review.

Note that some organizations also use either the trait analysis or tabula rasa technique to identify the most undesirable behaviors for purposes of creating a spectrum of the best and worst behaviors. Such a continuum is then used for pre-employment and post-employment evaluations.

The prerequisite for joyful involvement is aligned values. Without a clear and precise method for determining the behaviors that best suit values, there can be no joy. Joy cannot be found in an environment where values and tasks conflict.

A BARRIER-FREE WORKPLACE

How can anyone find joy in working when they keep running into obstacles to doing what they were hired (and what they desire) to do? I have interviewed hundreds of physicians and other clinical caregivers. One question I always ask of these groups is, "When are you at your best, and what is your more rewarding time here?" The answer is always a variation of this statement: "When I am allowed to use my skills to help patients."

Eliminating obstacles to high performers who display behaviors that reflect the corporate values is the key to creating joy in work (assuming that trust, respect, and pride are already in place). Analyzing the barriers is necessary and is quite simple to perform. As with the process of converting values to behaviors, there are two methods to analyze barriers: force field analysis (complex, but produces rich data) and high value, easy to do.

Force Field Analysis

Force field analysis (see Figure 5.1) is an organizational development technique that is useful in moving an organization forward. The first step in the process is to create a vision. Second, identify all the reasons (or driving forces) to move toward that vision. Third, list the current restraining forces that will cause the vision to fail. These restraining

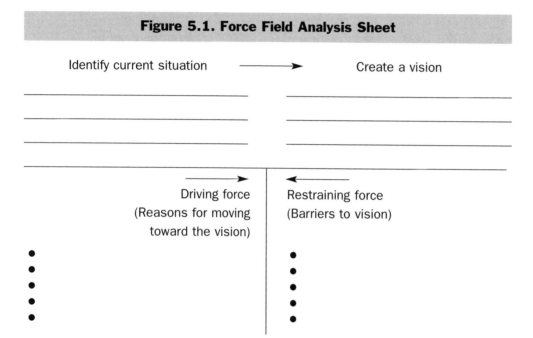

Figure 5.1. Force Field Analysis Sheet

Identify current situation   ⟶   Create a vision

⟶
Driving force
(Reasons for moving
toward the vision)

⟵
Restraining force
(Barriers to vision)

- •
- •
- •
- •
- •

- •
- •
- •
- •
- •

forces are the barriers, which can be classified into three:

1. *Personal:* barriers imbedded in someone's personality
2. *Interpersonal:* barriers of communication, decision making, and other interactions between people
3. *Structural:* barriers of doing business such as human resources policies, site location, and so on

Once the barriers are identified, only three things can be done: accept them, reduce their effects, or eliminate them. Figure 5.2 is a grid that is helpful in sorting the barriers

within their classifications.

Action plans (see Figure 5.3 on page 46) are necessary to eliminate the barriers. The sequence of managed-change intervention should be as follows: (1) eliminate structural barriers, (2) focus on interpersonal barriers that can be eradicated, (3) minimize structural barriers, and (4) target interpersonal barriers that can be reduced. The logic for such an intervention is to take action against those domains farthest from the ego (or the personal)—that is, structural and interpersonal. Eliminating structural barriers and reducing interpersonal barriers create a positive behavioral contagion or a ripple effect,

Figure 5.2. Grid for Sorting Barriers

Weighted Themes

Driving Force	Restraining Force
•	•
•	•
•	•
•	•
•	•
•	•

Barrier Classification

Personal

Eliminate	Reduce	Accept

Interpersonal

Eliminate	Reduce	Accept

Structural

Eliminate	Reduce	Accept

which alters the personal barriers that were identified during the brainstorming part of force field analysis.

High Value, Easy to Do
This technique again starts with a small group of high performers who are asked to list all of the barriers to joyful work. These barriers are written on a flip chart and are numbered. Each participant is then asked to vote on the two barriers that, if removed, would have the greatest positive impact on work. The resultant

Figure 5.3. Action Plan Sheet

Action Plan #1 — 30 days

- Who?_____

- What?_____

- When?_____

- How is success evaluated?_____

Action Plan #1 — 60 days

- Who?_____

- What?_____

- When?_____

- How is success evaluated?_____

Action Plan #1 — 90 days

- Who?_____

- What?_____

- When?_____

- How is success evaluated?_____

Figure 5.4. Personal Contract for Change

I, (Name) _____

promise to _____

_____

_____

These changes will be performed by

_____

I need to work with the following people if I am to fulfill this contract:

_____

_____

_____

list is the "high value" barriers. This high-value list is also numbered, and participants are asked to vote on one barrier from the list that is the easiest to remove or reduce. The second vote ends with 1 to 3 "high value, easy to do" targets.

Whether you use the force field analysis or the high value, easy to do method, the next step is to create a change plan for each target. A change plan has four components: (1) target, (2) accountabilities, (3) timeline, and (4) metrics.

A personal contract for change (see Figure 5.4) is often a good tool for ensuring that individual staff are involved in the change process.

CONCLUSION

Kelly Mather (2005), CEO at Sutter Lakeside Hospital in Lakeport, California, is a very creative, dynamic, and people-focused leader. When asked about how she creates joyful involvement in work among her staff, Mather states,

"I consistently survey the staff for their barriers and issues and then successfully reduce the barriers as often as possible. I meet with each department four times per year to ask them about what is working and what obstacles are interfering with work. Every staff person attending is asked to speak about [his or her] concerns, expectations, and ideas for improvement.

My job is to communicate, identify barriers, fix problems, and communicate the fix—and then start over." Mather adds, "[I] agree that reducing barriers allows for more joy. Isn't personal flexibility and reasonable expectations of yourself and others also a requirement for joy in work?"

All leaders spend a lot of time in self-reflection and personal development. It is here that healthcare leaders find joy in helping others be the best they can be for the good of the organizational mission.

Joy in work is the highest level of performance that a leader can create in the organization. It sits on top of the deeper dimensions of trust, respect, and pride. Alignment to the corporate culture and no unnecessary barriers are the formula for creating and building joy. Converting values to behaviors and barrier reduction are two processes that leaders often engage in with the help of high performers in the organization.

Leaders use the values-to-behaviors technique to strengthen the corporate culture as well as to hire and promote the professionals who are most aligned with the values of that culture. Engaging staff in barrier reduction allows them to take control of many of the issues that interfere with their performance.

REFERENCES

Atchison, T. A. 1990. *Turning Health Care Leadership Around: Cultivating Inspired, Empowered, and Loyal Followers*. San Francisco: Jossey-Bass.

———. 2001. "Striking a Balance." *Trustee* 54 (7): 28, 32.

———. 2002. "What is Corporate Culture?" *Trustee* 55 (4): 11.

———. 2004. *Followership: A Practical Guide to Aligning Leaders and Followers*. Chicago: Health Administration Press.

Atchison, T. A., and J. S. Bujak. 2002. *Leading Transformational Change: The Physician-Executive Partnership*. Chicago: Health Administration Press.

Csikszentmihalyi, M. 1994. *The Evolving Self: A Psychology for the Third Millennium.* New York: Harper Perennial.

Lambert, M., III. 2005. Personal communication with the author.

Mather, K. 2005. Personal communication with the author.

May, E. L. 2005. "Recruiting the Right Management Team for Organizational Transparency." *Healthcare Executive* 20 (4): 22–24, 26.

EXERCISE: Joy Inventory

Rate yourself (or have your staff evaluate you) on the following items.
5 = strongly agree; 4 = agree; 3 = sometimes agree; 2 = disagree;
1 = strongly disagree

1. My job fits my personality.

2. I like my coworkers.

3. We anticipate problems.

4. I feel like my work is important to the mission.

5. Time goes quickly at work.

6. At the end of the day, I feel tired—but it's a good tired.

7. I am happy with my work situation.

8. I am encouraged to identify barriers and solutions to my boss.

9. My work is challenging.

10. I often experience joy at work.

CHAPTER 6

The X Factor:
Synergy

Leaders who have the X factor translate individual parts into something unique and valuable.

Finding meaning in work. Finding joy in doing. Finding pride in accomplishment. These three statements are the purpose of this book.

Healthcare is a unique industry. People do not choose to spend their time, energy, and money in a hospital, or any healthcare facility, as they do willingly in other industries. Those who elect to work in healthcare are special in that they make themselves available to help those who do not want to be there. The challenge for healthcare leadership today is to keep the spirit of caring alive while trying to accommodate the often-faceless business aspects of the industry. This book presents a model designed to ensure that the caring infrastructure that defines healthcare is strong regardless of the vagaries of the marketplace. Too often, the infrastructure of trust, respect, pride, and joy are sacrificed on the altar of economic performance and short-sighted goals. ▶

The first five chapters of this book are linear, giving a framework of the multilayered deeper dimensions, offering methods for change, and laying out the outcomes: If you listen, trust develops; if you reward and recognize, respect results; if you challenge appropriately, pride is instilled; and if you knock down barriers to performance, joy happens. This model, however, has a fifth element—synergy. This bridge between the intangibles of trust, respect, pride, and joy and the tangibles of business, clinical, and regulation elements is very complicated.

Synergy is the X factor—the unknown that converts the four dimensions into a powerful force. Leaders who display this dynamic are alchemists—they transmute individual parts into something unique and valuable. It is that special dynamic that is difficult to define, is impossible to teach, but is very obvious when present.

The *Scott Foresman Advanced Dictionary* (1997) defines synergy as "the combined action of different agents or organs, producing a greater effect than the sum of the various individual actions." Leaders are able to create trust, respect, pride, and joy and then leverage these elements into a culture that is vital, is energizing, is self-corrective, and supports the organization's business, clinical, and regulatory realities. Leaders inspire the infrastructure in a way that produces synergy so that the tangibles can be managed.

The dictionary is a good place to start to understand the concept of synergy. However, this book will be remiss if it did not mention several healthcare leaders who consistently demonstrate the elusive synergy concept. Their words do a better job of explaining how synergy works. The leaders highlighted below are among the many who work hard at striking a balance between the art and science of healthcare. These leaders represent different types of hospitals (rural, tertiary, for-profit, and not-for-profit) and different regions in the United States.

SYNERGISTIC LEADERS

The X factor is defined by the spirit, not by the resume.

1. Chris Dadlez (2005), FACHE, president and CEO of Saint Francis Hospital and Medical Center in Hartford, Connecticut, explains that his X factor comes from this:

"Desire to create a work environment wherein individuals feel secure; where they can voice their opinion and ideas openly. I am here, quite simply, to stimulate others to be their best."

Dadlez believes that his desire "to help those who help those in need begins with selecting talented people who are nurturing and supportive, and, especially, do not put their ego needs first. But who enjoy helping others."

2. Bruce Jensen (2005), FACHE, president and CEO of St. Luke's Wood River Medical Center in Ketchum, Idaho, thinks that his X factor

"goes back to my roots and how I was raised. My underlying belief is that all people have an important role in life. I value everyone and feel that my role is to provide opportunities for each person to reach their potential. I don't know everything, but by building a team, I can learn how to help them help others. Each day is truly exciting to me. I love helping people make a difference."

3. David P. Engel (2005), trustee and immediate past chair of Christus

Spohn Health System in Corpus Christi, Texas, is called unique by Kathy McDonagh (2005), Ph.D., FACHE, the president and CEO of Christus Spohn, because "In any situation that David leads, those involved always leave that situation (regardless of the difficulty) feeling better than when they arrived." Engel explains that the X factor is a combination of

"a clear picture and strong passion . . . . I am able to picture in my mind what needs to be accomplished—I get a very clear picture. And I feel blessed that I am able to help others see the picture. Sometimes in working with others, the picture is altered, but always for the better. I am confident about moving forward because I believe in people. The X factor for me is a combination of seeing a picture and communicating passionately, while listening to the ideas, needs, and desires of others."

4. Rick Seidler (2005), FACHE, president and CEO of Allen Health System in Waterloo, Iowa, believes that the X factor that produces synergy is

"completely personal . . . [and] most obvious when I engage

others passionately about the importance of . . . producing the highest-quality outcomes for the people who need and count on us for care. I try to talk about our families and how we would want them cared for. Sure we run a business, but it is an incredibly personal business."

5. Jay Cox (2005), CHE, president and CEO of Tuomey Health System in Sumter, South Carolina, reasons that "the X factor is all about relationships." Cox periodically hosts "Leadership Advances" with his senior executives, physician leaders, and trustees. These leadership sessions always start with a sunrise walk on the beach. Such walks remind the participants about the importance of remembering that we are first people who share a great many good things. For Cox, the walks are an important part of the X factor because

"People who lead a healthcare organization must create a bond with those who deliver care. It's relationships first—not the issues. Years from now, no one will remember the specific topic or problem we worked on, but they will always remember the walks on the beach. Relationships are *how* we move forward and are much more relevant than *what* we do to move forward."

LESSONS FROM LEADERS WITH THE X FACTOR

1. Respect the past, live in the present, and have a clear picture of the future.
2. Appreciate people.
3. Get excited for others when they maximize their potential.
4. Strong egos are better than big egos.
5. Demonstrate and live the concept of servant leadership (see Greenleaf 2002).
6. Love your job.
7. Balance healthcare's human and business variables.
8. Learn for life.
9. Do not be afraid to do the right thing as opposed to the easy or popular thing.
10. Be and stay humble (see Atchison 2004).

REFERENCES

Atchison, T. A. 2004. *Followership: A Practical Guide to Aligning Leaders and Followers.* Chicago: Health Administration Press.

Cox, J. 2005. Personal communication with the author.

Dadlez, C. 2005. Personal communication with the author.

Engel, D. 2005. Personal communication with the author.

Greenleaf, R. 2002. *The Servant-Leadership: A Journey into the Nature of Legitimate Power and Greatness.* Mahwah, NJ: Paulist Press.

Jensen, B. 2005. Personal communication with the author.

McDonagh, K. 2005. Personal communication with the author.

EXERCISE: Work Group Inventory

Think of your work group. Place an "x" between the two ranges below to best describe how you currently view that work group.

Trust. . . . . Suspicion

Respect. . . . . Fear

Pride . . . . Anger

Joy. . . . . Apathy

Synergy . . . . Entropy

Suggested Reading List

Annison, M., and J. S. Bujak. 1998. *Trust Matters: How Doctors, Board Members and Health Care Executives Can Work Together Effectively*. San Diego: The Governance Institute, The Medical Leadership Forum.

Atchison, T. A. 1990. *Turning Health Care Leadership Around: Cultivating Inspired, Empowered, and Loyal Followers*. San Francisco: Jossey-Bass.

———. 1999. "The Myths of Employee Satisfaction." *Healthcare Executive* 14 (2): 18–23.

———. 2001. "Striking a Balance." *Trustee* 54 (7): 28, 32.

———. 2002. "What is Corporate Culture?" *Trustee* 55 (4): 11.

———. 2003. "Exposing the Myths of Employee Satisfaction." *Healthcare Executive* 18 (3): 20–26.

———. 2004. *Followership: A Practical Guide to Aligning Leaders and Followers*. Chicago: Health Administration Press.

Atchison, T. A., and J. S. Bujak. 2002. *Leading Transformational Change: The Physician-Executive Partnership*. Chicago: Health Administration Press.

Bennis, W., and B. Nanus. 1985. *Leaders: The Strategies for Taking Charge*. New York: HarperCollins.

Berwick, D. 2005. "The Importance and Paucity of Trust in Today's Healthcare System." *Trustee* 58 (4): 32.

Bracey, H. 2002. *Building Trust: How to Get It! How to Keep It!* Taylorsville, GA: HB Artworks, Inc.

Collins, J. 2001. *Good to Great: Why Some Companies Make the Leap and Others Don't*. New York: HarperCollins.

Csikszentmihalyi, M. 1994. *The Evolving Self: A Psychology for the Third Millennium*. New York: Harper Perennial.

———. 2003. *Good Business: Leadership, Flow, and the Making of Meaning*. New York: Penguin Books.

Frankl, V. 1983. *Man's Search for Meaning* (Revised and Updated). New York: Pocket Books.

Greenleaf, R. 2002. *The Servant-Leadership: A Journey into the Nature of Legitimate Power and Greatness*. Mahwah, NJ: Paulist Press.

Katzenbach, J. R. 2003. *Why Pride Matters More Than Money: The Power of the World's Greatest Motivational Force*. New York: Crown Business.

Kotter, J. P., and D. S. Cohen. 2002. *The Heart of Change*. Boston: Harvard Business School.

May, E. L. 2005. "Recruiting the Right Management Team for Organizational Transparency." *Healthcare Executive* 20 (4): 22–24, 26.

Rogers, R. W. 1999. *The Psychological Contract of Trust: Trust Development in the 90's Workplace*. Pittsburgh, PA: Development Dimensions International.

Schein, E. R. 1997. *Organizational Culture and Leadership, Second Edition*. San Francisco: Jossey-Bass.

Shore, D. A. 2005. *The Trust Prescription for Healthcare*. Chicago: Health Administration Press.

ABOUT THE AUTHOR

Tom Atchison, Ed.D., is president and founder of The Atchison Consulting Group, Inc. (now Atchison Consulting, LLC). Since 1984, Dr. Atchison has consulted with healthcare organizations on managed-change programs, teambuilding, and leadership development. He also has consulted to the military, healthcare vendors, and government agencies on the intangible aspects of healthcare. His consulting practice focuses on measuring and managing the intangibles that drive change. Typically, he consults to senior executives, managers, trustees, and physician leaders.

Dr. Atchison presents to thousands of healthcare professionals each year on the elements of effective organizations. He has written and has been featured in a number of articles and audiotapes and videotapes about motivation, managed change, teambuilding, and leadership. He is the author of *Turning Healthcare Leadership Around, Leading Transformational Change: The Physician-Executive Partnership*, and *Followership: A Practical Guide to Aligning Leaders and Followers*.

Dr. Atchison's expertise in healthcare is built on more than 30 years of experience in a variety of management positions in healthcare institutions and organizations. Dr. Atchison is a Member of the American College of Healthcare Executives. He earned his doctorate degree in human resources development from Loyola University of Chicago.

ACKNOWLEDGMENTS

As I have mentioned in previous books, I find writing to be a difficult journey from the initial idea to the final product. For me, this is an impossible journey to take alone. Many people helped me stay focused and moving forward. For example, the wonderful staff at HAP—Janet Davis, Audrey Kaufman, Kaye Muench, and Jane Williams—must be recognized for their encouragement, support, and, especially, their patience (I don't always make the deadlines!).

My family, especially my wife, deserves a big thank you for understanding why I needed to write rather than join them at an outing. Finally, the office staff—Letty, Elia, and Marty—need to be noted for their loyalty and their ability to keep "all of the balls in the air" and still help me put this book together. Of these three stars, Letty Saldivar needs special thanks. She is a unique individual who always seems to find a way to do the best job in the shortest amount of time. Her intelligence, patience, and friendship are the main reasons that this book and hundreds of other yearly projects we take on look and sound so good.

A common practice is to dedicate a book to one or more persons for their unique and special characteristics. This book is therefore dedicated to the hundreds of thousands of very caring healthcare professionals who come to work every day for the single purpose of helping others. In an industry that is constantly bombarded by economic, legal, and regulatory pressures, the beauty of these great people is that they still find meaning, pride, and joy in each day.

Thank you all.

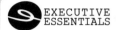
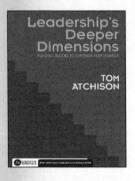 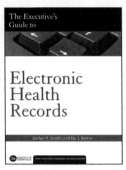 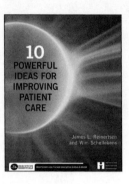 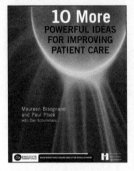 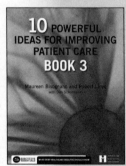
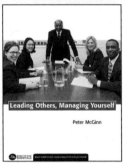 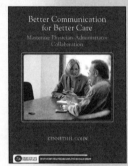
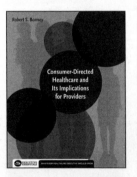 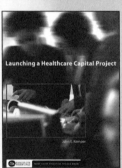
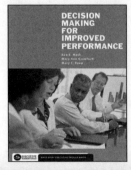 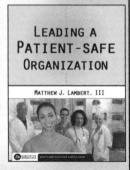
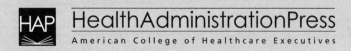